REVITALIZE YOUR HEALTH:

A COMPREHENSIVE GUIDE TO WEIGHT LOSS AND

TYPE 2 DIABETES REVERSAL THROUGH

INTERMITTENT FASTING AND LOW-CARB LIVING

Contents

About me

My name is Dwayne Burks-Green, and at age 35, I was confronted with a diagnosis of type 2 diabetes. Juggling long work hours, a diet saturated with processed foods, irregular exercise, excessive alcohol consumption, and overweight, I found myself at a health crossroad. Determined not to rely solely on medications, I delved into books and scoured YouTube for solutions to transform my health. Within a mere 6 months, I successfully reversed a myriad of health issues such as high blood pressure, diabetes, erectile dysfunction, and alcohol dependency, shedding over 30 pounds in the process. This book serves as a testament to my journey and details the precise steps I took to achieve this remarkable turnaround.

Dear Readers, before embarking on any methods detailed in this book, I strongly advise consulting a physician to ensure they align with your individual health needs and circumstances."

Introduction

Welcome to "Revitalize Your Health: A Comprehensive Guide to Weight Loss and Type 2 Diabetes Reversal Through Intermittent Fasting and Low-Carb Living." In the bustling landscape of health and wellness, there exists a powerful synergy between lifestyle choices, nutrition, and disease management. This guide is crafted as a roadmap for those seeking transformative changes in their health, focusing on two potent tools: intermittent fasting and a low-carb lifestyle.

In a world marked by sedentary habits, processed foods, and rising health concerns, it's crucial to navigate through the noise and discover practical, evidence-based approaches to rejuvenate both body and mind. The journey to weight loss and the reversal of Type 2 diabetes requires more than fleeting trends; it demands a holistic understanding and commitment to sustainable lifestyle modifications.

Throughout the following chapters, we will delve into the intricacies of Type 2 diabetes, exploring its origins and the pivotal role that obesity plays in its development. We will unravel the science behind intermittent fasting, shedding light on its potential benefits for weight management and blood sugar control. Simultaneously, we'll explore the transformative impact of adopting a low-carb lifestyle, dismantling misconceptions and offering practical insights on how to seamlessly incorporate it into daily life.

As we embark on this journey together, we'll address the vital connection between physical activity, fasting, and low-carb living, illustrating how a well-rounded approach can amplify results. This guide is not just about short-term fixes; it's about instilling lasting habits that promote overall well-being, creating a sustainable foundation for a healthier, more vibrant life.

Whether you're grappling with the challenges of Type 2 diabetes or simply seeking a comprehensive guide to weight loss and improved health, "Revitalize Your Health" is designed to empower you. It's a call to action, an invitation to reclaim control over your health narrative. Let's embark on this transformative journey together, uncovering the keys to revitalizing your health and achieving lasting well-being.

Chapter 1:

Understanding Type 2 Diabetes

Introduction to Type 2 diabetes: Definition, prevalence, and impact on health.

Type 2 diabetes, a metabolic disorder characterized by elevated blood sugar levels, stands as a significant health challenge in our modern society. As we delve into the intricacies of this condition, understanding its definition, prevalence, and impact on health is crucial for anyone seeking to navigate the landscape of wellness.

Definition:

Type 2 diabetes, often referred to as adult-onset diabetes, is a chronic condition that affects the way the body processes glucose. Glucose, a sugar derived from the food we consume, serves as the primary energy source for cells. Insulin, a hormone produced by the pancreas, facilitates the entry of glucose into cells. In individuals with Type 2 diabetes, the body either doesn't produce enough insulin or doesn't use it effectively, leading to an accumulation of glucose in the bloodstream.

This disruption in glucose regulation can result in a range of symptoms, including increased thirst, frequent urination, fatigue, and slow wound healing. Left unmanaged, Type 2 diabetes can contribute to more severe complications such as cardiovascular disease, kidney dysfunction, and nerve damage.

Prevalence:

The prevalence of Type 2 diabetes has reached alarming levels worldwide, transforming it into a global health concern. Sedentary lifestyles, poor dietary choices, and an aging population have contributed to the escalating rates of diagnosis. According to the World Health Organization (WHO), approximately 90% of all diabetes cases are Type 2, highlighting the urgency to address its roots and implement effective prevention and management strategies.

In many societies, the prevalence of Type 2 diabetes is intertwined with the rising tide of obesity. Excess body weight, especially around the abdomen, significantly increases the risk of developing insulin resistance, a hallmark of Type 2 diabetes. As we explore the impact of lifestyle changes on diabetes management, recognizing the symbiotic relationship between obesity and Type 2 diabetes becomes imperative.

Impact on Health:

Beyond its immediate symptoms, Type 2 diabetes casts a long shadow on overall health. The persistent elevation of blood sugar levels can lead to systemic inflammation and damage bloodvessels, increasing the risk of heart disease and stroke. Additionally, the kidneys and nerves are susceptible to harm, emphasizing the multisystemic impact of this condition.

The profound implications of Type 2 diabetes extend beyond physical health, affecting emotional well-being and quality of life. Managing a chronic condition requires vigilance, lifestyle adjustments, and often a complex medication regimen. As we navigate the chapters ahead, we will explore not only how to manage and potentially reverse Type 2 diabetes but also how toenhance overall health and vitality.

In the pursuit of optimal well-being, understanding the fundamentals of Type 2 diabetes sets the stage for informed decision-making and empowers individuals to take control of their health narrative. Let us now embark on a journey to unravel the transformative power of intermittent fasting and low-carb living in the quest to revitalize health and conquer Type 2 diabetes.

Causes and risk factors: Explore the factors contributing to the development of Type 2 diabetes.

The development of Type 2 diabetes is a multifaceted interplay between genetic, lifestyle, and environmental factors. Unraveling the intricate web of causes and risk factors is essential for understanding the origins of this prevalent metabolic disorder and devising effective strategies for prevention and management.

Genetic Predisposition:

Genetics plays a pivotal role in the susceptibility to Type 2 diabetes. Individuals with a family history of diabetes are at an increased risk, suggesting a genetic predisposition that can influence how the body regulates glucose. Specific gene variants related to insulin production and glucose metabolism contribute to this hereditary component. However, genetics alone does not determine the onset of Type 2 diabetes; environmental factors and lifestyle choices also play crucial roles.

Insulin Resistance:

A hallmark of Type 2 diabetes is insulin resistance, where cells become less responsive to the effects of insulin. This impaired response hinders the efficient uptake of glucose from the bloodstream into cells, leading to elevated blood sugar levels. The exact mechanisms behind insulin resistance are complex and can be influenced by factors such as obesity, physical inactivity, and certain hormonal imbalances.

Obesity and Body Composition:

Excess body weight, particularly abdominal obesity, is a significant contributor to the development of Type 2 diabetes. Adipose tissue, especially around the abdomen, releases inflammatory substances that can interfere with insulin signaling. The link between obesity and diabetes underscores the importance of weight management as a preventive and therapeutic measure.

Physical Inactivity:

A sedentary lifestyle and lack of regular physical activity are independent risk factors for Type 2 diabetes. Exercise enhances insulin sensitivity, allowing cells to better respond to insulin and effectively utilize glucose. In contrast, prolonged periods of Inactivity contributes to weight gain, exacerbates insulin resistance, and increases the likelihood of developing diabetes.

Dietary Choices:

The modern diet, often characterized by excessive consumption of processed foods, refined sugars, and high-calorie, low-nutrient options, is implicated in the rising rates of Type 2 diabetes. Diets rich in refined carbohydrates and saturated fats can contribute to obesity, insulin resistance, and metabolic dysfunction. On the contrary, adopting a balanced, nutrient-dense diet can play a pivotal role in preventing and managing Type 2 diabetes.

Age and Ethnicity:

Age is a non-modifiable risk factor, with the risk of Type 2 diabetes increasing with advancing age. Additionally, certain ethnic groups, such as African Americans, Hispanics, Native Americans, and Asian Americans, are more prone to developing diabetes. The reasons behind these ethnic disparities are multifaceted, involving genetic, lifestyle, and socioeconomic factors.

Understanding the causes and risk factors of Type 2 diabetes is the foundation for developing targeted interventions. As we delve deeper into this comprehensive guide, we will explore how lifestyle modifications, including intermittent fasting and a low-carb living approach, can effectively address and mitigate these contributing factors, offering a pathway toward diabetes reversal and improved overall health.

The link between obesity and diabetes: Understanding the connection and its implications.

In the intricate tapestry of metabolic health, the link between obesity and Type 2 diabetes is a crucial thread that weaves through the landscape of modern health challenges. Understanding this connection is paramount to addressing the root causes of diabetes and developing effective strategies for prevention and management.

The Adipose Tissue Influence:

Obesity, especially visceral or abdominal obesity, serves as a significant contributor to the development of Type 2 diabetes. Adipose tissue, commonly known as fat, is not just an inert storage depot but an active endocrine organ. In individuals with excess body weight, particularly around the abdomen, adipose tissue secretes pro- inflammatory substances and hormones that can disrupt normal metabolic processes, leading to insulin resistance.

Insulin Resistance and Its Escalation:

Insulin resistance, a hallmark of Type 2 diabetes, occurs when cells become less responsive to the effects of insulin. As adipose tissue expands due to obesity, it releases free fatty acids into the bloodstream. Elevated levels of circulating fatty acids can interfere with insulin signaling, hindering the ability of cells to efficiently take up glucose. This sets in motion a vicious cycle where insulin resistance contributes to weight gain, and obesity exacerbates insulin resistance, creating a self-perpetuating loop.

Inflammatory Factors:

Obesity is associated with a state of chronic low-grade inflammation. Adipose tissue releases inflammatory cytokines and substances such as tumor necrosis factor-alpha (TNF-") and interleukin-6 (IL-6). This chronic inflammation further impairs insulin signaling, contributing to the progression from insulin resistance to full-blown Type 2 diabetes.

Inflammation also plays a role in the development of other diabetes-related complications, including cardiovascular disease.

Implications for Diabetes Prevention and Management:

Recognizing the intricate link between obesity and Type 2 diabetes holds significant implications for both prevention and management strategies. Weight loss and maintenance of a healthy body weight are key components in preventing the onset of diabetes in individuals at risk. Lifestyle modifications that focus on reducing body fat, especially around the abdomen, can positively impact insulin sensitivity and lower the risk of diabetes.

In the context of diabetes management, addressing obesity becomes an essential component of an effective treatment plan. Weight loss interventions, including dietary changes, increased physical activity, and behavioral modifications, can lead to improved glycemic control and a reduction in the need for diabetes medications. Moreover, as we explore in subsequent chapters, incorporating intermittent fasting and adopting a low-carb lifestyle can synergistically enhance the effectiveness of weight management efforts.

Understanding the profound connection between obesity and Type 2 diabetes allows individuals to make informed choices about their health. As we navigate the journey to revitalize health through intermittent fasting and low-carb living, acknowledging and addressing the impact of obesity on diabetes is a pivotal step toward achieving lasting wellness.

Important lifestyle changes: Emphasize the role of lifestyle modifications in managing and potentially reversing Type 2 diabetes.

In the realm of Type 2 diabetes management, the significance of lifestyle changes cannot be overstated. Lifestyle modifications stand as the cornerstone of an effective, holistic approach, offering individuals the power to not only manage their condition but potentially reverse its course. By embracing a proactive and intentional shift in habits, individuals can exert considerable influence over their health outcomes, fostering lasting well-being and vitality.

Breaking the Cycle of Insulin Resistance:

Lifestyle changes play a pivotal role in breaking the cycle of insulin resistance, a central feature of Type 2 diabetes. Adopting healthier eating habits and engaging in regular physical activity can lead to weight loss and a reduction in visceral fat, directly impacting insulin sensitivity. This, in turn, allows cells to more efficiently respond to insulin, facilitating the uptake of glucose and helping to restore normal metabolic function.

Improving Blood Sugar Control:

A key objective in managing Type 2 diabetes is achieving and maintaining optimal blood sugar levels. Lifestyle changes, particularly those related to dietary choices and physical activity, have a direct impact on glycemic control. By choosing nutrient-dense, low-carb foods and incorporating regular exercise, individuals can help regulate blood sugar levels, reducing the reliance on medications and mitigating the risk of diabetes-related complications.

Enhancing Cardiovascular Health:

Type 2 diabetes is often associated with an increased risk of cardiovascular diseases. Lifestyle modifications, such as adopting a heart-healthy diet and engaging in regular exercise, not only support diabetes management but also contribute to overall cardiovascular health. These changes can positively influence blood pressure, and cholesterol levels, and reduce the risk of heart-related complications, providing a holistic approach to well- being.

Sustainable Weight Management:

Obesity is a significant risk factor for Type 2 diabetes, and lifestyle changes are instrumental in achieving and maintaining a healthy weight. By promoting sustainable weight loss through a balanced diet and increased physical activity, individuals can reduce the burden on their metabolic systems, aiding in the management and potential reversal of diabetes.

Psychological Well-being:

The impact of lifestyle changes extends beyond physical health, influencing psychological well-being. Adopting a health-focused lifestyle can empower individuals, boost self-esteem, and reduce stress levels.

Stress management techniques, mindfulness practices, and adequate rest becomes integral components of a holistic approach to managing Type 2 diabetes.

Long-Term Sustainability:

One of the distinguishing features of lifestyle changes is their potential for long-term sustainability. Unlike quick-fix solutions, transformative modifications become ingrained habits, woven into the fabric of daily life. This sustainability is key to the successful management and potential reversal of Type 2 diabetes, providing a foundation for lasting health and resilience.

As we embark on the journey of revitalizing health through intermittent fasting and low-carb living, it is essential to recognize the transformative power of lifestyle changes. This guide is notjust about managing diabetes; it's about empowering individuals to reclaim control over their health narratives and fostering enduring well-being through intentional and sustainable choices. The journey to diabetes reversal begins with a commitment to lifestyle changes—a commitment that holds the promise of a healthier, more vibrant life.

Chapter 2 :

Exploring Intermittent Fasting

Definition and types of intermittent fasting: Break down different fasting methods, such as 16/8, 5:2, and alternate-day fasting.

Intermittent fasting has gained widespread popularity as a powerful tool for weight management, metabolic health, and potential benefits for individuals with Type 2 diabetes. Understanding the definition and various types of intermittent fasting is pivotal for those embarking on this transformative journey.

Definition of Intermittent Fasting:

Intermittent fasting is not a diet in the traditional sense but rather an eating pattern that cycles between periods of eating and fasting. Unlike conventional diets that prescribe specific foods to eat or avoid, intermittent fasting focuses on when to eat. The primary goal is to create extended periods of fasting, allowing the body to tap into stored energy reserves and undergo various metabolic processes associated with health and well-being.

Types of Intermittent Fasting:

1. 16/8 Method (Time-Restricted Eating):

- **Description:** Also known as time-restricted eating, the 16/8 method involves daily fasting for 16 hours and restricting eating to an 8-hour window. For example, one might eat between 12:00 pm and 8:00 pm, followed by a 16-hour fasting period until the next day at 12:00 pm.

- **Benefits:** This method is relatively easy to incorporate into daily life and aligns with the body's natural circadian rhythm. It can aid in weight management, improve insulin sensitivity, and promote fat utilization during fasting periods.

2. 5:2 Diet:

- **Description:** The 5:2 diet involves regular eating for five days a week and restricting caloric intake to around 500-600 calories on two non-consecutive days. These fasting days can be chosen based on personal preference, but they should not be consecutive.

- **Benefits:** This method offers flexibility while still providing the potential benefits of intermittent fasting. It may promote weight loss, improve metabolic health, and contribute tobetter blood sugar control.

3. Alternate-Day Fasting:

- **Description:** In alternate-day fasting, individuals alternate between days ofregular eating and days of either complete fasting or significant caloric restriction (around 500 calories). This method can be more challenging due to the alternating nature of fasting and feasting.

- **Benefits:** Alternate-day fasting may result in more significant weight loss and improvements in metabolic markers. However, it requires careful adherence to avoid overcompensating on non-fasting days.

4. Eat-Stop-Eat:

- **Description:** This method involves a 24-hour fast once or twice a week. For instance, an individual might fast from dinner one day to dinner the next day, resulting in a 24-hour fasting period.

- **Benefits:** Eat-Stop-Eat can be effective for weight loss and may contribute to improved insulin sensitivity. However, adherence to a full-day fast can be challenging for some individuals.

5. Warrior Diet:

- **Description:** The Warrior Diet involves eating small amounts of raw fruits and vegetables during the day and consuming one large meal at night, typically within a 4-hour eating window.

- **Benefits:** This method combines short periods of undereating with a longer daily fasting window. It may be suitable for those who prefer a more lenient approach to intermittent fasting.

It's essential to note that the effectiveness and suitability of each intermittent fasting method can vary from person to person. Choosing the right approach often depends on individual preferences, lifestyle, and health goals. As we navigate through this comprehensive guide, we'll explore how these intermittent fasting methods can be seamlessly integrated into a low-carb lifestyle to maximize their potential benefits for weight loss and Type 2 diabetes management.

Scientific research on intermittent fasting: Summarize key studies highlighting thepotential benefits for weight loss and blood sugar control.

The surge of interest in intermittent fasting has prompted numerous scientific studies to explore its impact on various aspects of health, including weight management and blood sugar control. Summarizing key findings from these studies sheds light on the potential benefits and provides evidence-based insights into the efficacy of intermittent fasting.

Weight Loss and Fat Reduction:

A randomized ***controlled trialpublished in JAMA Internal Medicine (2017):***

- **Key Findings:** This study compared the effects of time-restricted eating (similar to the 16/8 method) with a regular eating schedule. The results indicated that participants in the time-restricted eating group experienced significant weight loss, primarily attributed to a reduction in overall caloric intake and improved fat metabolism during fasting periods.

A review published in Obesity Reviews (2015):

- **Key Findings:** This comprehensive review analyzed various intermittent fasting approaches, including alternate-day fasting and the 5:2 diet. The synthesis of multiple studies suggested that intermittent fasting is an effective strategy for promoting weight loss and reducing body fat, with participants generally achieving comparable or even greater weight loss than traditional calorie-restricted diets.

Blood Sugar Control and Insulin Sensitivity:

A study published in Cell Metabolism (2018):

- **Key Findings:** This study investigated the effects of time-restricted eating on insulin sensitivity and glucose metabolism. The results demonstrated improved insulin sensitivity and lower fasting insulin levels in participants practicing time-restricted eating. This suggests that intermittent fasting may have positive effects on blood sugar control and reduce the risk of insulin resistance.

A randomized ***controlled trial published in Diabetes Care (2017):***

- **Key Findings:** This study examined the impact of alternate-day fasting on individuals with Type 2 diabetes. The findings revealed significant improvements in glycemic control, including reductions in fasting glucose levels and insulin resistance. Participants also experienced beneficial changes in body weight and cardiovascular risk factors.

A meta-analysis published in PLOS ONE (2015):

- **Key Findings:** This meta-analysis synthesized data from various intermittent fasting studies and explored its effects on glycemic control. The analysis suggested that intermittent fasting interventions, including time-restricted eating and alternate-day fasting, were associated with improved insulin sensitivity and reduced fasting glucose levels.

Cardiometabolic Health:

A review published in Circulation Research (2019):

- **Key Findings:** This comprehensive review examined the impact of intermittent fasting on cardiovascular health. The review highlighted potential benefits, such as improvements in blood pressure, lipid profiles, and inflammation. These findings suggest that intermittent fasting may contribute to overall cardiometabolic health beyond its effects on weight and blood sugar.

A study published in The American Journal of Clinical Nutrition (2019):

- **Key Findings:** This study investigated the effects of intermittent fasting on cardiovascular risk factors in individuals with obesity. The results indicated reductions in various risk factors, including blood pressure and triglyceride levels. These cardiovascular improvements add to the growing body of evidence supporting the potential holistic benefits of intermittent fasting.

While scientific research on intermittent fasting continues to evolve, these key studies underscore the promising potential of intermittent fasting for weight loss, blood sugar control, and overall metabolic health. As we delve deeper into this comprehensive guide, we will explore how incorporating intermittent fasting into a low-carb lifestyle can synergistically enhance these benefits, offering a multifaceted approach to revitalizing health and managing Type 2 diabetes.

How intermittent fasting affects insulin sensitivity: Explore the physiological changes that occur during fasting and their impact on Type 2 diabetes.

Intermittent fasting, characterized by cycles of eating and fasting, has emerged as a compelling strategy for managing Type 2 diabetes by influencing insulin sensitivity. Delving into the physiological changes that occur during fasting sheds light on how intermittent fasting can positively impact insulin resistance and contribute to the management ofthis metabolic disorder.

1. Improved Insulin Sensitivity:

- **Insulin Sensitivity Defined:** Insulin sensitivity refers to how effectively cells respond to insulin's signal, allowing them to absorb glucose from the bloodstream. In individuals with Type 2 diabetes, insulin sensitivity is often impaired, leading to elevated blood sugar levels.

- **Physiological Changes:** Intermittent fasting promotes improved insulin sensitivity by reducing the frequency and duration of elevated blood sugar levels. During fasting periods, the body relies on stored energy, encouraging cells to become more responsive to insulin when foodis consumed.

2. Regulation of Blood Glucose Levels:

- **Normalizing Blood Sugar Levels:** Intermittent fasting helps regulate blood glucose levels by preventing constant spikes and providing periods ofrest for insulin-producing cells in the pancreas.

- **Physiological Changes:** Fasting periods lead to a reduction in circulating glucose, prompting the body to tap into glycogen stores for energy. This process helps maintain blood sugar levels within a more stable range, preventing the continuous strain on insulin-producing cells.

3. Enhanced Fat Metabolism:

- **Reducing Fat Accumulation:** Excessive fat accumulation, particularly around abdominal organs, contributes to insulin resistance. Intermittent fasting encourages the utilization of storedfats for energy.

- **Physiological Changes:** During fasting, the body enters a state of ketosis, where it relies on ketones produced from fat breakdown for energy. This shift in fuel utilization not only aids in weight loss but also reduces fat accumulation, positively impacting insulin sensitivity.

4. Cellular Repair and Autophagy:

- **Cellular Cleansing Mechanisms:** Autophagy, the cellular process of recycling damaged or dysfunctional components, is upregulated during fasting. This process contributes to cellular repair and maintenance.

- **Physiological Changes:** Autophagy helps remove damaged mitochondria and other cellular structures, promoting overall cellular health. This can play a role in reducing inflammation and enhancing insulin sensitivity.

5. Reduction in Inflammatory Markers:

- **Chronic Inflammation and Insulin Resistance:** Chronic inflammation is closely linked to insulin resistance. Intermittent fasting has been shown to reduce inflammatory markers, contributing to improved insulin sensitivity.

- **Physiological Changes:** Fasting periods suppress inflammatory pathways, leading to a decrease in proinflammatory substances. This anti-inflammatory effect contributes to a more favorable metabolic environment.

6. Hormonal Regulation:

- **Impact of Hormones on Insulin Sensitivity:** Hormones such as insulin, cortisol, and glucagon play key roles in regulating glucose metabolism. Intermittent fasting influences the balance of these hormones.

- **Physiological Changes:** Fasting periods lead to reduced insulin levels and increased glucagon secretion, promoting glucose release from the liver. This hormonal shift helps maintain blood sugar levels while enhancing insulin sensitivity.

Understanding how intermittent fasting affects insulin sensitivity provides valuable insights into its potential benefits for individuals with Type 2 diabetes. By promoting physiological changes that support better glucose control and metabolic health, intermittent fasting emerges as a promising strategy in the comprehensive approach to managing and potentially reversing Type 2 diabetes. As we continue our exploration, we will uncover how combining intermittent fasting with a low-carb lifestyle amplifies these physiological benefits, offering a synergistic approach to revitalizing health.

Addressing common concerns and misconceptions about intermittent fasting.

Intermittent fasting, with its rising popularity, has sparked a multitude of questions and concerns. While this eating pattern has shown promising health benefits, addressing common misconceptions is essential for individuals considering incorporating intermittent fasting into their lifestyles. Let's explore and clarify some of the prevalent concerns surrounding intermittent fasting.

1. Fear of Starvation:

- **Misconception:** One common concern is the fear of starvation or malnutrition during fasting periods.

- **Clarification:** Intermittent fasting is not about depriving the body of essential nutrients. Instead, it involves cycles of eating and fasting, allowing the body to tap into stored energy reserves. Adequate hydration and balanced nutrition during eating windows ensure that nutritional needs are met.

2. Impact on Metabolism:

- **Misconception:** Some worry that intermittent fasting might slow down metabolism, making weight management more challenging.

- **Clarification:** Research suggests that intermittent fasting can boost metabolism. During fasting, the body's metabolic rate may increase, and the shift towards fat utilization for energy can support weight loss efforts.

3. Energy Levels and Productivity:

- **Misconception:** Concerns often arise about energy levels and productivity during fasting periods.

- **Clarification:** While there may be an adjustment period as the body adapts to intermittent fasting, many individuals report improved energy levels and mental clarity. Proper hydration and balanced meals during eating windows help support sustained energy.

4. Adequacy of Nutrition:

- **Misconception:** Some worry that intermittent fasting may lead to nutritional deficiencies.

- **Clarification:** Intermittent fasting can be implemented with a focus on balanced, nutrient-dense meals during eating windows. A well-rounded diet, including a variety of food groups, helps ensure that nutritional needs are met.

5. Feasibility for Different Lifestyles:

- **Misconception:** People often wonder if intermittent fasting is feasible for those with demanding schedules or specific dietary requirements.

- **Clarification:** Intermittent fasting is flexible and can be adapted to various lifestyles. It is customizable, allowing individuals to choose the fasting method that aligns with their preferences, schedules, and dietary needs.

6. Suitability for Everyone:

- **Misconception:** There's a perception that intermittent fasting is not suitable for everyone,particularly those with certain health conditions.

- **Clarification:** While intermittent fasting may not be suitable for everyone, its potential benefits extend to a broad range of individuals. Consulting with a healthcare professional before starting any fasting regimen is crucial, especially for those with pre-existing health conditions.

7. Need for Strict Adherence:

- **Misconception:** Some believe that intermittent fasting requires rigid adherence to specific schedules.

- **Clarification:** Intermittent fasting can be flexible. While consistency is beneficial, occasional adjustments based on social events or personal preferences are acceptable without negating potential benefits.

Addressing these concerns and misconceptions can help individuals make informed decisions about incorporating intermittent fasting into their lives. It's crucial to approach intermittent fasting with a balanced perspective, understanding that its feasibility and impact can vary among individuals. As with any significant lifestyle change, consulting with a healthcare professional ensures that intermittent fasting aligns with individual health goals and requirements.

Chapter 3 :

The Low-Carb Lifestyle

Introduction to low-carb diets: Define what constitutes a low-carb diet and its historical context.

In the intricate landscape of dietary choices, low-carb diets have emerged as a compelling approach to nutrition, capturing attention for their potential benefits in weight management, blood sugar control, and overall health. This introduction aims to define what constitutes a low-carb diet and delve into its historical context, shedding light on the foundations of this dietary philosophy.

Defining a Low-Carb Diet:

A low-carb diet, as the name suggests, is characterized by a reduced intake of carbohydrates, a primary macronutrient found in foods such as grains, legumes, fruits, and starchy vegetables. Instead, the focus is placed on obtaining energy from alternative sources, such as proteins and fats. The primary goal is to minimize the consumption of simple carbohydrates and refined sugars, which can lead to fluctuations in blood sugar levels and contribute to weight gain.

Typically, a low-carb diet encourages the consumption of nutrient-dense foods like lean proteins, non-starchy vegetables, healthy fats, and moderate portions of whole grains. The emphasis is on selecting carbohydrates with a lower glycemic index to promote more stable blood sugar levels and sustained energy throughout the day.

Historical Context of Low-Carb Diets:

The roots of low-carb diets can be traced back to the mid-19th century, gaining notable prominence in the 20th century with the advent of various diet trends. One of the earliest proponents of low-carb eating was William Banting, an English undertaker, who published a pamphlet titled "Letter on Corpulence" in 1863. Banting advocated for reducing the intake of bread, sugar, beer, and potatoes, a dietary approach that mirrored the principles of contemporary low-carb diets.

In the latter half of the 20th century, Dr. Robert Atkins played a pivotal role in popularizing low-carb diets with the publication of his groundbreaking book, "Dr. Atkins' Diet Revolution" in 1972. The Atkins Diet promoted a significant reduction in carbohydrate intake while encouraging the consumption of protein and fats. Dr. Atkins' approach sparked a widespread reevaluation of traditional dietary guidelines and contributed to the ongoing discourse surrounding the impact of carbohydrates on health.

Over the years, variations of low-carb diets have emerged, including the ketogenic diet, South Beach Diet, and Paleo diet, each with its unique emphasis on carbohydrate restriction and specific food choices. The resurgence of interest in low-carb diets in recent decades reflects a growing recognition of their potential benefits, not only for weight management but also for metabolic health and chronic disease prevention.

As we navigate through the chapters of this guide, we will delve deeper into the principles, benefits, and practical aspects of incorporating a low-carb lifestyle. Understanding the historical context and evolution of low-carb diets provides a foundation for exploring how this dietary approach can be seamlessly integrated into modern lifestyles for optimal health and well-being.

Benefits of a low-carb lifestyle: Discuss the positive effects on weight loss, blood sugar regulation, and overall health.

Embracing a low-carb lifestyle transcends mere dietary choices; it represents a holistic approach to wellness with far-reaching benefits. Let's explore the positive effects of a low-carb lifestyle, delving into how it can nurture weight loss, regulate blood sugar levels, and foster overall health.

1. Efective Weight Loss:

• **Metabolic Shift:** One of the primary benefits of a low-carb lifestyle is its efficacy in promoting weight loss. By reducing the intake of carbohydrates, the body shifts its primary energy source from glucose to stored fats, initiating a process known as ketosis. This metabolic shift encourages the body to utilize fat energy stores, aiding in weight loss and the reduction of body fat.

• **Appetite Regulation:** Low-carb diets often contribute to improved appetite regulation. The consumption of protein and healthy fats helps create a sense of satiety, reducing overall calorie intake. This can be particularly advantageous for those seeking sustainable weight loss without the constant struggle of dealing with hunger pangs.

2. *Blood Sugar Regulation:*

- **Stabilized Blood Glucose Levels:** A hallmark benefit of a low-carb lifestyle is its positive impact on blood sugar regulation. By minimizing the intake of high-glycemic carbohydrates, the diet helps prevent sharp spikes and crashes in blood glucose levels. This stability is crucial for individuals with Type 2 diabetes or those at risk of developing insulin resistance.

- **Improved Insulin Sensitivity:** Low-carb diets have been associated with improved insulin sensitivity. By reducing the demand for insulin in response to carbohydrate intake, cells become more responsive to the hormone. This can contribute to better blood sugar control and reduce the risk of developing Type 2 diabetes.

3. *Cardiovascular Health:*

- **Lowered Risk Factors:** Adopting a low-carb lifestyle has been linked to improvements in various cardiovascular risk factors. This includes reductions in triglyceride levels, an increase in high-density lipoprotein (HDL or "good" cholesterol), and improvements in blood pressure. These factors collectively contribute to a lower risk of heart disease and related complications.

- **Inflammation Reduction:** Chronic inflammation is a contributing factor to cardiovascular diseases. Low-carb diets, especially those rich in anti-inflammatory foods, have shown potential in reducing systemic inflammation. This anti-inflammatory effect further supports Cardiovascular health.

4. Enhanced Mental Clarity and Energy Levels:

- **Steady Energy:** The avoidance of blood sugar spikes and crashes associated with high-carb diets contributes to more stable energy levels throughout the day. By relying on fats and ketones for energy, individuals often report improved mental clarity and sustained focus.

- **Potential Cognitive Benefits:** Some research suggests that a low-carb lifestyle may have cognitive benefits. The brain can efficiently utilize ketones for energy, and anecdotal evidence indicates that individuals on low-carb diets experience enhanced cognitive function.

5. Reduced Risk of Chronic Diseases:

- **Prevention of Metabolic Syndrome:** Metabolic syndrome, characterized by a cluster of conditions including obesity, high blood pressure, and insulin resistance, is associated with an increased risk of chronic diseases. A low-carb lifestyle has shown promise in preventing and managing metabolic syndrome and reducing the risk of diabetes and cardiovascular diseases.

- **Influence on Cancer Risk:** Emerging research suggests that a low-carb lifestyle may have implications for cancer prevention. While more studies are needed, the potential link between reduced carbohydrate intake and a lower risk of certain cancers is a topic of ongoing investigation.

Embracing a low-carb lifestyle goes beyond short-term dietary changes; it embodies a comprehensive approach to well-being. By nurturing weight loss, regulating blood sugar, and fostering overall health, individuals can unlock the transformative potential of this lifestyle. As we navigate through the following chapters, we will explore practical strategies for incorporating a low-carb approach into daily life, empowering individuals to reap the manifold benefits and embark on a journey to revitalized health.

Types of low-carb diets: Explore popular approaches like ketogenic, Atkins, and Mediterranean diets.

The realm of low-carb diets offers a diverse array of approaches, each with its unique principles and emphases. Exploring popular low-carb diets, such as the ketogenic, Atkins, and Mediterranean diets, unveils the rich tapestry of options available for those seeking to embrace a carbohydrate-conscious lifestyle.

1. Ketogenic Diet:

- **Principles:** The ketogenic diet, often referred to as keto, is characterized by a significant reduction in carbohydrate intake and a notable increase in the consumption of fats. The primary goal is to induce a state of ketosis, where the body shifts from utilizing glucose as its primary fuel to burning ketones, derived from fats.

- **Food Choices:** A typical ketogenic diet includes high-fat foods such as avocados, nuts, seeds, oils, and fatty fish. Moderate protein intake is allowed, while carbohydrates are limited to a minimal amount, usually around 20-50 grams per day.

- **Benefits:** The ketogenic diet is renowned for its efficacy in promoting rapid weight loss and improving blood sugar control. It has also shown promise in managing neurological conditions such as epilepsy and providing sustained energy levels.

2.Atkins Diet:

- **Phases:** The Atkins Diet is structured in phases, each with its unique carbohydrate allowance. It begins with a strict induction phase, limiting carbs to jumpstart weight loss, followed by phases that gradually reintroduce more carbohydrates while still promoting weight maintenance.

- **Carb Restriction:** While the initial phases of the Atkins Diet involve significant carb restriction, the later phases aim to find an individual's "Critical Carbohydrate Level for Maintenance" (CCLM), where weight is maintained without gaining or losing.

- **Food Choices:** The Atkins Diet emphasizes whole foods, including proteins, healthy fats, and non-starchy vegetables. Processed foods and sugars are restricted throughout the diet.

3. Mediterranean Diet:

- **Principles:** The Mediterranean diet is renowned for its emphasis on whole, nutrient-dense foods inspired by the traditional dietary patterns of countries bordering the Mediterranean Sea. While not strictly a low-carb diet, it naturally tends to be lower in carbohydrates compared to typical Western diets.

- **Food Choices:** The diet includes an abundance of fruits, vegetables, nuts, seeds, legumes, whole grains, and healthy fats such as olive oil.

Fish and lean proteins are also staples, while red meat is consumed in moderation.

- **Benefits:** The Mediterranean diet is associated with various health benefits, including improved cardiovascular health, weight management, and reduced risk of chronic diseases. Its moderate approach to carbohydrates makes it a sustainable and flexible dietary choice.

4. Low Carb High Fat (LCHF) Diet:

- **Principles:** The Low Carb High Fat (LCHF) diet shares similarities with the ketogenic diet but allows for a more flexible carbohydrate intake. It focuses on reducing carbs while incorporating healthy fats and maintaining a moderate protein intake.

- **Food Choices:** The LCHF diet encourages the consumption of whole foods, including meats, fish, eggs, nuts, seeds, dairy, and non-starchy vegetables. It limits processed foods, sugars, and grains.

- **Benefits:** The LCHF diet is praised for its potential to support weight loss, improve metabolic health, and provide sustained energy levels. It offers flexibility, allowing individuals to find a carbohydrate intake that suits their needs and goals.

5. Eco-Atkins Diet:

- **Principles:** The Eco-Atkins diet is a plant-based variation of the traditional Atkins Diet. It maintains a low-carb approach while emphasizing plant-based protein sources.

- **Food Choices:** The diet includes plant-based proteins such as legumes, tofu, and seitan, along with non-starchy vegetables, nuts, and seeds. It limits the consumption of animal products and encourages the inclusion of plant-based fats.

- **Benefits:** The Eco-Atkins diet aims to provide the benefits of a low-carb approach while aligning with vegetarian or vegan dietary preferences. It may offer advantages in terms of weight management and cardiovascular health.

Navigating these types of low-carb diets allows individuals to choose an approach that aligns with their preferences, health goals, and lifestyle. Whether seeking the rapid ketosis of a ketogenic diet, the structured phases of Atkins, the balanced principles of the Mediterranean diet, the flexibility of LCHF, or the plant-based focus of Eco-Atkins, the spectrum of low carb options provides a versatile toolkit for those embarking on a journey toward improved health and vitality. As we progress through this guide, we will delve deeper into practical strategies for adopting and sustaining a low-carb lifestyle, empowering individuals to embrace the approach that resonates most with their unique needs.

Practical tips for transitioning to a low-carb lifestyle: Provide guidance on grocery shopping, meal planning, and dining out.

Embarking on a low-carb lifestyle involves not just a shift in dietary choices but also a reorientation of your approach to food. Practical tips for transitioning seamlessly to a low-carb lifestyle can make the journey enjoyable and sustainable. Let's explore guidance on grocery shopping, meal planning, and dining out to set you on the path to success.

1. Grocery Shopping:

- **Focus on Whole Foods:** Prioritize whole, unprocessed foods when filling your cart. Fresh vegetables, lean proteins, nuts, seeds, and healthy fats should form the foundation of your grocery list.

- **Read Labels:** Pay attention to food labels to identify hidden sugars and excessive carbohydrate content in processed items. Opt for products with minimal added sugars and refined carbohydrates.

- **Stock Up on Low-Carb Staples:** Ensure your pantry is well-stocked with low-carb staples such as olive oil, coconut oil, herbs and spices, nut flours, and alternative sweeteners (if desired). These ingredients provide the foundation for diverse and satisfying low-carb meals.

- **Choose Quality Proteins:** Select high-quality proteins like grass-fed meats, poultry, fish, and eggs. These proteins not only contribute to satiety but also offer essential nutrients.

2. Meal Planning:

- **Plan Balanced Meals:** Aim for a well-balanced plate with a mix of non-starchy vegetables, proteins, and healthy fats. This combination provides essential nutrients while keeping carb intake in check.

- **Prepare in Advance:** Consider preparing meals in advance, especially ifyou have a busy schedule. Batch cooking on weekends can save time during the week and ensure you always have a low-carb option available.

- **Explore** Low-Carb **Recipes:** The internet is a treasure trove of delicious low-carb recipes. Experiment with new dishes to keep your meals exciting and varied. Websites, blogs, and cook books dedicated to low-carb cooking offer a plethora of ideas.

- **Portion Control:** While low-carb eating is about the quality of the foods you consume, portion control is still crucial for managing overall calorie intake. Be mindful of serving sizes to support your health and weight management goals.

3. *Dining Out:*

- **Check Menus in Advance:** When planning to dine out, review the menu online beforehand. This allows you to identify low-carb options and make informed choices, reducing the temptation to stray from your dietary goals at the moment.

- **Opt for Grilled or Roasted Proteins:** Choose grilled or roasted proteins like chicken, fish, or steak when dining out. These options are often lower in added carbohydrates compared to breaded or fried alternatives.

- **Request Modifications:** Don't hesitate to request modifications to accommodate your low-carb preferences. Ask for substitutions, such as a side salad instead of fries, or extra vegetables in place of starch-heavy sides.

- **Beware of Hidden Carbs:** Be mindful of sauces, dressings, and marinades that may contain hidden sugars or high carbohydrate content. Ask for these items on the side, allowing you to control your intake.

4. *Stay Hydrated:*

- **Drink Water:** Adequate hydration is crucial, especially when transitioning to a low-carb lifestyle. Water helps support digestion, alleviate cravings, and maintain overall health. Carry a water bottle with you to ensure you stay hydrated throughout the day.

- **Limit Sugary Beverages:** Cut back on sugary beverages, including sodas and sweetened juices. Opt for water, herbal teas, or black coffee as low-carb alternatives.

- **Consider Electrolytes:** As your body adjusts to reduced carbohydrate intake, you may experience changes in electrolyte levels. Consider incorporating electrolyte-rich foods or supplements to support overall well-being.

Transitioning to a low-carb lifestyle is a gradual process, and these practical tips can smooth the way. By prioritizing whole foods, planning your meals, navigating dining-out scenarios thoughtfully, and staying hydrated, you'll find that adopting a low-carb approach becomes an enjoyable and sustainable part of your daily life. As you integrate these strategies, you'll discover a wealth of delicious and satisfying low-carb options that contribute not only to your health goals but also to a renewed sense of well-being.

Chapter 4 :

Integrating Exercise with Fasting and Low-Carb Lifestyle

Importance of exercise in diabetes management: Discuss the role of physical activity in improving insulin sensitivity and promoting weight loss.

Physical activity is a cornerstone of effective diabetes management, offering a range of benefits that extend beyond cardiovascular health. Exercise plays a crucial role in improving insulin sensitivity and promoting weight loss, key components in managing and preventing Type 2 diabetes. Understanding the importance of incorporating regular physical activity into one's lifestyle can empower individuals on their journey toward better health.

1. Improving Insulin Sensitivity:

• **Insulin and Glucose Dynamics:** Insulin sensitivity refers to how effectively cells respond to insulin's signal, allowing them to absorb glucose from the bloodstream. In individuals with Type 2 diabetes, insulin sensitivity is often impaired, leading to elevated blood sugar levels.

• **Enhanced Glucose Uptake:** Exercise stimulates the muscles to take up glucose from the blood for energy, independent of insulin. This process improves insulin sensitivity, helping cells become more responsive to insulin over time. As a result, blood sugar levels are better regulated.

- **Long-Term Benefits:** Regular physical activity can have long-lasting effects on insulin sensitivity. Consistent exercise helps create a positive cycle, where improved insulin sensitivity leads to better blood sugar control, making it easier for the body to manage glucose levels effectively.

2. Promoting Weight Loss and Maintenance:

- **Energy Expenditure:** Exercise is a potent tool for weight management, as it contributes to increased energy expenditure. Physical activity burns calories, helping individuals achieve a calorie deficit, which is essential for weight loss.

- **Building Lean Muscle Mass:** Resistance training and other forms of exercise contribute to the development of lean muscle mass. Muscle tissue has a higher metabolic rate than fat tissue, meaning that the more muscle one has, the more calories one burns even at rest. This can support weight loss and weight maintenance over time.

- **Enhancing Metabolism:** Regular physical activity can boost metabolism, making it more efficient at utilizing nutrients for energy. This metabolic enhancement, coupled with a balanced diet, aids in weight loss and contributes to overall well-being.

3. Managing Blood Sugar Levels:

- **Post-Exercise Glucose Uptake:** Exercise has an immediate impact on blood sugar levels. After physical activity, muscles are more receptive to glucose uptake, leading to a temporary reduction in blood sugar. This effect can be particularly beneficial for individuals with diabetes,helping to manage post-meal glucose spikes.

• **Aiding Medication Effectiveness:** For those using medications to manage diabetes, exercise complements the action of these drugs. Improved insulin sensitivity and better blood sugar control achieved through regular physical activity can enhance the effectiveness of diabetes medications.

4. *Cardiovascular Health:*

• **Reducing Cardiovascular Risk:** Cardiovascular health is a significant concern for individuals with diabetes. Regular exercise contributes to reducing the risk of cardiovascular diseases by improving heart function, lowering blood pressure, and managing cholesterol levels.

• **Enhanced Blood Circulation:** Exercise promotes better blood circulation, ensuring that organs and tissues receive an adequate supply of oxygen and nutrients. This is crucial for overall health and can help prevent complications associated with diabetes.

5. *Psychological Well-Being:*

• **Stress Reduction:** Managing stress is essential for individuals with diabetes, as stress can impact blood sugar levels. Exercise acts as a natural stress reliever, promoting mental well-being and contributing to overall emotional balance.

- **Improved Mood:** Physical activity stimulates the release of endorphins, often referred to as "feel-good" hormones. This can lead to an improved mood, reduced symptoms of anxiety and depression, and a positive outlook on life - crucial elements in diabetes management.

Incorporating regular exercise into a diabetes management plan is a powerful strategy for enhancing insulin sensitivity, promoting weight loss, and improving overall health. Individuals with diabetes should consult with their healthcare team to tailor an exercise regimen that aligns with their individual needs, considering factors such as current fitness level, health status, and any existing complications. By making physical activity an integral part of daily life, individuals can take proactive steps toward optimal diabetes management and a healthier, more vibrant lifestyle.

Best exercises for individuals with Type 2 diabetes: Tailor exercises to accommodate various fitness levels and preferences.

Physical activity is a cornerstone of effective Type 2 diabetes management, offering a spectrum of benefits from improved blood sugar control to enhanced cardiovascular health. When crafting an exercise routine for individuals with Type 2 diabetes, it's crucial to consider various fitness levels, preferences, and any potential health limitations. Let's explore a range of exercises that can be tailored to accommodate different needs, fostering a personalized approach to physical activity.

1.Aerobic Exercises:

- **Walking:** Walking is a low-impact exercise suitable for individuals of all fitness levels. It can be adapted to various environments, from outdoor trails to indoor malls, and serves as an excellent starting point for those new to regular physical activity.

- **Cycling:** Whether using a stationary bike or cycling outdoors, this activity provides an effective cardiovascular workout. It's gentle on the joints, making it suitable for individuals with varying fitness levels and joint concerns.

- **Swimming:** Swimming is a full-body workout that's easy on the joints. It offers the benefits of cardiovascular exercise while providing resistance for muscle strengthening. Water aerobics or water walking are also excellent options for those seeking variety.

- **Dancing:** Engaging in dance, whether through classes or at-home routines, combines exercise with enjoyment. Dance is adaptable to different fitness levels, offering a fun way to improve cardiovascular health.

2.Strength Training:

- **Bodyweight Exercises:** Exercises like squats, lunges, push-ups, and planks, utilize body weight for resistance. These exercises can be modified to accommodate different fitness levels, making them suitable for beginners and those with varying degrees of strength.

- **Resistance Band Workouts:** Resistance bands provide a portable and versatile option for strength training. They offer controlled resistance, helping individuals build muscle without the need for heavy weights.

• **Weightlifting:** For those comfortable with weightlifting, incorporating light to moderate weights can enhance muscle strength and improve overall metabolic health. Workouts can be tailored to individual preferences and goals.

3. Flexibility and Balance Exercises:

• **Yoga:** Yoga is beneficial for improving flexibility, balance, and overall well-being. It comes in various forms, from gentle Hatha yoga to more dynamic Vinyasa or Power yoga, allowing individuals to choose a style that aligns with their fitness level.

• **Tai Chi:** Tai Chi is a low-impact exercise that combines slow, flowing movements with deep breathing. It enhances balance, flexibility, and mindfulness, making it suitable for individuals of all ages and fitness levels.

• **Stretching Routines:** Incorporating stretching exercises into a routine promotes flexibility and joint health. Simple stretches can be adapted to accommodate different fitness levels and can be done at home or in a group setting.

4. High-Intensity Interval Training (HIIT):

• **Adapted HIIT Workouts:** High-intensity interval Training involves short bursts of intense activity followed by periods of rest. Individuals can tailor HIIT workouts to their fitness level, adjusting the duration and intensity of exercise intervals.

- **Consultation with Healthcare Professionals:** Before starting a high-intensity exercise program, individuals should consult with their healthcare team to ensure it is suitable for their health status and any existing conditions.

5. Group Activities:

- **Group Fitness Classes:** Participating in group fitness classes, whether in person or virtually, can add a social element to exercise. Options like Zumba, spinning, or group strength training classes offer a supportive environment for individuals with varied fitness levels.

- **Walking Groups:** Joining a walking group provides social interaction along with the benefits of walking. It's a simple yet effective way to stay motivated and enjoy physical activity with others.

When designing an exercise routine for individuals with Type 2 diabetes, it's essential to consider individual preferences, fitness levels, and any existing health conditions. Before initiating any new exercise program, consulting with healthcare professionals is paramount. They can provide personalized guidance, considering factors such as medications, blood sugar levels, and potential complications. With a tailored approach to physical activity, individuals with Type 2 diabetes can enjoy the diverse benefits of exercise while maintaining optimal health and well-being.

Timing exercise with intermittent fasting: Explore optimal workout times in relation to fasting periods for maximum benefits.

The combination of intermittent fasting and exercise can be a powerful strategy for individuals seeking optimal health, weight management, and improved insulin sensitivity. When considering the timing of exercise in relation to intermittent fasting, careful planning can enhance the benefits of both practices. Let's explore how strategic workout timing during fasting periods can maximize the advantages of this synergistic approach.

1. Exercising in the Fasted State:

• **Morning Workouts:** For individuals practicing time-restricted eating or daily intermittent fasting, engaging in exercise during the morning hours can align with the fasting period. This allows individuals to leverage the benefits of fasting-induced metabolic changes, including increased fat utilization for energy.

• **Enhanced Fat Burning:** Exercising in the fasted state may enhance the body's ability to burn stored fat for fuel. With reduced glycogen stores from the overnight fast, the body relies on fat as a primary energy source during exercise.

• **Improved Insulin Sensitivity:** Fasted workouts have shown the potential to improve insulin sensitivity. Combining intermittent fasting with morning exercise may create a synergistic effect, amplifying the positive impact on blood sugar control.

2. Post-Workout Nutrient Timing:

- **Breaking the Fast with Nutrient-Rich Foods:** Following a workout, individuals can strategically break their fast with a nutrient-dense meal. This post-workout meal can include a combination of protein, healthy fats, and carbohydrates to replenish glycogen stores and support muscle recovery.

- **Protein Intake:** Prioritizing protein intake after exercise is crucial for muscle repair and growth. Including lean proteins such as poultry, fish, tofu, or legumes in the post-workout meal supports these processes.

- **Carbohydrates for Glycogen Replenishment:** Including complex carbohydrates, such as whole grains or fruits, helps replenish glycogen stores depleted during fasting and exercise. This contributes to sustained energy levels and aids in recovery.

3. Afternoon or Evening Workouts:

- **Flexibility in Exercise Timing:** While morning workouts align with fasting periods, afternoon or evening workouts can also be beneficial. For individuals with different schedules or preferences, the key is to ensure that the fasting window still provides ample time for recovery post-exercise.

- **Hydration and Electrolytes:** Staying hydrated throughout the fasting period and during workouts is essential. Adequate water intake, along with electrolyte-rich beverages if needed, supports optimal performance and recovery.

4. Individual Considerations:

- **Listen to Your Body:** The optimal timing for exercise during intermittent fasting can vary among individuals. Listening to your body and choosing a workout time that aligns with your energy levels, preferences, and daily routine is crucial for long-term adherence.

- **Consideration for Health Conditions:** Individuals with certain health conditions, such as diabetes, cardiovascular issues, or metabolic disorders, should consult with healthcare professionals before implementing a fasting and exercise regimen. Personalized advice ensures that the chosen approach aligns with individual health needs.

5. Balancing Intensity and Duration:

- **Tailoring Exercise Intensity:** High-intensity workouts during fasting periods may not be suitable for everyone. Balancing exercise intensity with individual fitness levels and fasting duration ensures a sustainable and safe approach.

- **Moderate Exercise Duration:** While longer, moderate-intensity workouts can contribute to increased fat utilization, it's essential to avoid overtraining during fasting periods. Striking a balance that supports overall well-being is key.

Integrating exercise into an intermittent fasting routine requires thoughtful consideration of individual preferences and health factors. Whether opting for morning workouts during the fasting window or choosing alternative times, the goal is to align exercise with fasting periods to maximize the synergistic benefits of both practices. Prioritizing recovery with nutrient-rich meals post-workout ensures that the body receives the essential elements for optimal health and performance. As with any lifestyle change, consulting with healthcare professionals provides personalized guidance, helping individuals tailor their approach to achieve their health and fitness goals.

Overcoming challenges: Address common obstacles and provide strategies to stay motivated and consistent with exercise.

Embarking on a fitness journey comes with its share of challenges, but overcoming obstacles is an integral part of achieving long-term success. Whether it's finding motivation, navigating time constraints, or dealing with setbacks, adopting effective strategies can help individuals stay motivated and consistent with their exercise routine. Let's explore common challenges and actionable solutions to ensure a resilient and sustainable approach to fitness.

1. Challenge: Lack of Motivation:

- **Solution:** Set Clear Goals: Define specific, measurable, and achievable fitness goals. Whether it's weight loss, improved endurance, or strength building, having a clear objective provides a sense of purpose and motivation.

- **Find Enjoyable Activities:** Engage in exercises or activities that you genuinely enjoy. Whether it's dancing, hiking, or playing a sport, finding enjoyment in your workouts makes it more likely that you'll stick with them.

- **Create a Support System:** Share your fitness journey with friends or join a fitness community. Having a support system can provide encouragement, accountability, and a sense of camaraderie.

2. Challenge: Time Constraints:

- **Solution: Prioritize and Schedule:** Treat exercise as a non-negotiable part of your routine. Prioritize your health by scheduling workouts just like any other commitment. Short, focused workouts can be effective and fit into busy schedules.

- **Optimize Time:** Combine activities where possible, such as walking or biking to work, taking the stairs, or doing quick, high-intensity workouts. Look for opportunities to incorporate movement throughout the day.

- **Break It Down:** If a full workout seems daunting, break it down into shorter sessions. Ten minutes of exercise multiple times a day can be just as effective as a longer session.

3. Challenge: Plateau in Progress:

- **Solution:** Change Up Your Routine: Plateaus are common in fitness, but they can be overcome by introducing variety into your routine. Try different exercises, change the intensity, or explore new workout formats to challenge your body in new ways.

- **Set Progressive Goals:** Continuously challenge yourself by setting new fitness goals. This could be increasing the intensity, duration, or frequency of your workouts. Gradual progression keeps your body adapting and prevents stagnation.

- **Celebrate Non-Scale Victories:** Focus on the positive changes beyond the scale, such as improved stamina, increased flexibility, or enhanced mood. Celebrating these victories reinforces the value of your efforts.

4. Challenge: Lack of Consistency:

- **Solution:** Establish a Routine: Consistency is key to seeing results. Establish a regular exercise routine by choosing specific days and times for your workouts. Treat these appointments with the same importance as any other commitment.

- **Start Small:** Building consistency is easier when you start with manageable goals. Begin with shorter, more frequent workouts and gradually increase the duration and intensity as your routine becomes more ingrained.

- **Be Flexible:** Life can be unpredictable, and schedules may change. Embrace flexibility and find alternative times or activities if your original plan is disrupted. The key is to keep moving forward.

5. Challenge: Lack of Confidence:

- **Solution:** Focus on Progress, Not Perfection: Shift your mindset from perfection to progress. Understand that everyone starts somewhere, and improvements take time. Celebrate small achievements and acknowledge your efforts.

- **Seek Guidance:** If you're unsure about exercises or form, consider seeking guidance from a fitness professional. Whether through a personal trainer or online resources, understanding proper techniques boosts confidence.

- **Surround Yourself with Positivity:** Surround yourself with positive influences, whether it's supportive friends, motivational quotes, or uplifting music. Building a positive environment can boost your confidence and outlook.

6. Challenge: Health Issues or Injuries:

- **Solution:** Consult with Healthcare Professionals: If you have health concerns or existing injuries, consult with healthcare professionals or fitness experts before starting a new exercise routine. They can provide guidance on safe and appropriate activities.

- **Modify Workouts:** If certain exercises are off-limits due to health issues or injuries, explore modified versions or alternative activities that accommodate your condition. Adaptability is key to maintaining a consistent routine.

- **Focus on Recovery:** Incorporate proper warm-up and cool-down routines into your workouts, and prioritize recovery strategies such as stretching, foam rolling, and adequate rest. A holistic approach to fitness includes caring for your body's recovery needs.

7. Challenge: Mental Health Struggles:

- **Solution:** Recognize the Mental Health Benefits: Regular exercise has proven mental health benefits, including stress reduction and mood enhancement. Acknowledge the positive impact that exercise can have on your overall well-being.

- **Choose Mindful Activities:** Engage in activities that promote mindfulness, such as yoga or meditation. These practices not only contribute to physical well-being but also provide mental clarity and stress relief.

- **Seek Professional Support:** If mental health challenges persist, consider seeking support from mental health professionals. Therapists or counselors can provide guidance and strategies to navigate mental health struggles in conjunction with your fitness journey.

Overcoming challenges in the realm of fitness requires a combination of determination, adaptability, and a positive mindset. By addressing common obstacles with strategic solutions, individuals can create a sustainable and enjoyable exercise routine that contributes to overall health and well-being. Remember that every step forward, no matter how small,brings you closer to your fitness goals.

Chapter 5 :

Creating a Comprehensive Approach for Maximum Results

Developing a personalized plan: Guide readers in crafting an individualized approach that combines intermittent fasting, a low-carb lifestyle, and exercise.

Embarking on a journey to improved health involves crafting a personalized plan that integrates key elements such as intermittent fasting, a low-carb lifestyle, and exercise. This comprehensive approach addresses various aspects of well-being, from metabolic health to sustainable weight management. Let's guide readers in developing an individualized plan that harmoniously combines these components, fostering a holistic approach to optimal health.

1. Assess Current Lifestyle and Health Status:

- **Reflect on Current Habits:** Begin by reflecting on your current lifestyle, dietary habits, and exercise routine. Identify patterns that support or hinder your health goals.

- **Consult with Healthcare Professionals:** Before making significant changes, consult with healthcare professionals, including a doctor or a registered dietitian. They can provide insights based on your health status and help tailor recommendations to your unique needs.

2. Define Clear Health Goals:

● **Set SMART Goals:** Establish Specific, Measurable, Achievable, Relevant, and Time-bound (SMART) health goals. Whether it's weight loss, improved blood sugar control, or increased physical fitness, clear objectives provide direction for your plan.

● **Prioritize Long-Term Well-Being:** While immediate results are gratifying, prioritize long-term well-being. Consider how your plan can contribute to sustained health improvements over time.

3. Integrate Intermittent Fasting:

● **Choose** a **Fasting Window:** Determine an intermittent fasting window that aligns with your lifestyle. Options include daily time-restricted eating (e.g.,16/8 method), alternate-day fasting, or modified fasting approaches.

● **Gradual Implementation:** If new to intermittent fasting, consider a gradual implementation. Start with a shorter fasting window and gradually extend it as your body adjusts.

4. Embrace a Low Carb Lifestyle:

● **Identify Carbohydrate Sources:** Assess your current carbohydrate sources and identify opportunities to replace refined carbs with whole, nutrient-dense options. Focus on non-starchy vegetables, lean proteins, healthy fats, and moderate portions of whole grains.

● **Experiment with Different Approaches:** Explore various low-carb diets, such as ketogenic, Atkins, or Mediterranean. Choose an approach that aligns with your preferences and is sustainable for your lifestyle.

5. Design an Exercise Routine:

- **Select Enjoyable Activities:** Choose exercises that you enjoy to enhance adherence. Whether it's walking, cycling, strength training, or group fitness classes, enjoyable activities increase the likelihood of long-term commitment.

- **Incorporate Variety:** Include a variety of exercises to target different muscle groups and aspects of fitness. This not only prevents monotony but also provides a comprehensive approach to overall health.

- **Consider Timing with Fasting:** If possible, align exercise with fasting periods. For instance, consider morning workouts during the fasting window to maximize fat utilization for energy.

6. Prioritize Adequate Sleep and Hydration:

- **Ensure Quality Sleep:** Quality sleep is integral to overall health. Prioritize sufficient and restful sleep, as it influences metabolism, hormone regulation, and overall well-being.

- **Stay Hydrated:** Adequate hydration supports various bodily functions, including digestion, metabolism, and exercise performance. Aim for a consistent intake of water throughout the day.

7. Monitor Progress and Adjust as Needed:

- **Regular Assessments:** Periodically assess your progress toward health goals. This can include monitoring weight, measuring fitness improvements, or tracking changes in blood sugar levels.

- **Be Flexible and Adaptive:** Recognize that individual needs and circumstances may evolve. Be flexible and open to adjusting your plan based on personal experiences, feedback from healthcare professionals, and evolving health goals.

8. Foster a Supportive Environment:

- **Seek Social Support:** Share your health journey with friends, family, or a supportive community. Having a network of encouragement can bolster motivation and provide valuable insights.

- **Celebrate Achievements:** Acknowledge and celebrate achievements, both big and small. This positive reinforcement contributes to a more positive mindset and reinforces your commitment tothe plan.

Crafting a personalized plan that seamlessly integrates intermittent fasting, a low-carb lifestyle, and exercise is a dynamic process. By assessing your current habits, defining clear health goals, and tailoring your approach to individual preferences and needs, you create a roadmap for sustained well-being. Remember that health is a holistic journey, and adopting a comprehensive plan allows you to navigate this path with intention, flexibility, and a focus on long-term vitality.

Monitoring progress: Discuss the importance of tracking weight, blood sugar and overall well-being to gauge success.

Embarking on a health journey that involves intermittent fasting, a low-carb lifestyle, and regular exercise is a commendable step towards overall well-being. To ensure the success of your personalized plan, monitoring progress becomes an integral aspect of the process. Keeping a close eye on key indicators such as weight, blood sugar levels, and overall well-being provides valuable insights, helping you make informed adjustments and celebrate your achievements along the way.

1. Weight Tracking:

- **Understanding Body Composition:** Monitoring changes in weight is a tangible way to gauge progress. However, it's essential to consider body composition, as fluctuations in muscle mass and fat distribution may impact overall weight.

- **Set Realistic Expectations:** Recognize that weight loss can occur at varying rates, and factors such as water retention, muscle gain, and hormonal changes may influence the numbers on the scale. Set realistic expectations and focus on overall well-being rather than solely on weight.

- **Consistent Measurement:** If tracking weight, aim to measure consistently, such as at the same time of day and under similar conditions. This provides a more accurate representation of your progress.

2. *Blood Sugar Level Monitoring:*

- **Understanding Glycemic Control:** For individuals incorporating intermittent fasting and a low-carb lifestyle to manage blood sugar levels, regular monitoring is crucial. Track fasting blood glucose levels and observe how dietary and lifestyle changes impact glycemic control.

- **Utilize Continuous Glucose Monitoring (CGM):** Continuous Glucose Monitoring devices offer a real-time view of blood sugar trends throughout the day. They can provide valuable insights into how dietary choices and fasting windows influence glucose levels.

- **Consult with Healthcare Professionals:** Interpretation of blood sugar data may require guidance from healthcare professionals. Regular discussions with your doctor or a registered dietitian can help refine your approach based on your individual responses.

3. *Overall Well-Being:*

- **Energy Levels:** Assess changes in energy levels and overall vitality. Increased energy, mental clarity, and improved mood are positive indicators that your health plan is contributing to your well-being.

- **Sleep Quality:** Track improvements in sleep quality. Quality sleep is essential for overall health, and positive changes in sleep patterns often accompany lifestyle modifications.

- **Mental and Emotional Well-Being:** Consider the impact on mental and emotional well-being. Reduced stress levels, improved focus, and a positive outlook are qualitative indicators of progress that extend beyond numerical measurements.

4. *Fitness and Exercise Performance:*

- **Strength and Endurance:** Gauge improvements in strength and endurance. Whether it's lifting heavier weights, running longer distances, or achieving new fitness milestones, these indicators showcase the positive impact of regular exercise.

- **Flexibility and Mobility:** Assess improvements in flexibility and mobility. Enhanced range of motion and reduced stiffness are indicative of positive changes in musculoskeletal health.

- **Recovery Time:** Monitor post-exercise recovery time. A reduction in soreness and faster recovery between workouts suggests improved fitness levels and adaptability.

5. *Celebrate Non-Scale Victories:*

- **Clothing Fit:** Pay attention to changes in how your clothes fit. Positive alterations in clothing size or fit can be indicative of body composition improvements.

- **Increased Physical Activity:** Celebrate achievements related to increased physical activity. Whether it's completing a challenging workout, participating in a new fitness class, or consistently hitting daily step goals, these victories contribute to overall success.

- **Nutritional Choices:** Acknowledge positive changes in dietary choices. The ability to make informed, health-conscious food decisions is a non-scale victory that supports long-term well-being.

6. Periodic Assessments and Adjustments:

- **Regular Check-Ins:** Schedule periodic check-ins to assess progress and make any necessary adjustments to your plan. Regular evaluations ensure that your health journey remains dynamic and responsive to your evolving needs.

- **Document Changes:** Keep a record of changes, both positive and areas for improvement. This documentation provides a comprehensive overview of your health journey and informs future decisions.

7. Seek Professional Guidance:

- **Consult Healthcare Professionals:** If facing challenges or uncertainties, seek guidance from healthcare professionals. Your doctor, registered dietitian, or fitness trainer can offer valuable insights and support tailored to your individual circumstances.

- **Medical Check-Ups:** Schedule regular medical check-ups to monitor overall health. These appointments provide an opportunity for comprehensive assessments and discussions about your health goals.

Monitoring progress is a holistic approach that extends beyond numerical values. While weight, blood sugar levels, and fitness milestones provide quantitative data, paying attention to qualitative improvements in overall well-being and lifestyle choices is equally crucial. By adopting a well-rounded monitoring strategy, you empower yourself to make informed decisions, celebrate achievements, and navigate your health journey with intention and adaptability.

Remember that progress is a dynamic process, and each step forward contributes to your ongoing success.

Potential setbacks and troubleshooting: Address common challenges and provide solutions for overcoming plateaus or difficulties.

Embarking on a health journey that involves intermittent fasting, a low-carb lifestyle, and regular exercise is undoubtedly rewarding, but it may come with its share of challenges. Recognizing potential setbacks and proactively troubleshooting them is essential for maintaining motivation and sustaining progress. Let's address common challenges and provide practical solutions to overcome plateaus or difficulties on your path to optimal health.

1. *Plateaus in Weight Loss:*

- **Evaluate Caloric Intake:** Assess your caloric intake and ensure you're still in a calorie deficit, especially if weight loss has plateaued. Adjust portion sizes, monitor snacking habits, and be mindful of hidden calories.

- **Vary Exercise Routine:** If exercising regularly, consider incorporating variety into your workout routine. The body may adapt to repetitive exercises, leading to a plateau. Try new activities, increase intensity, or explore different workout modalities.

- **Consult Healthcare Professionals:** If weight loss stalls despite consistent efforts, consult with healthcare professionals, including a registered dietitian or doctor, to rule out underlying factors and receive personalized guidance.

2. *Challenges with Consistency:*

- **Reassess Goals:** Reflect on your health goals and ensure they align with your current lifestyle and priorities. Adjust goals if necessary to make them realistic and achievable, fostering sustained motivation.

- **Establish Routines:** Develop consistent daily routines that integrate intermittent fasting, meal planning, and exercise. A structured schedule enhances adherence and minimizes decision fatigue.

- **Seek Social Support:** Share your health journey with friends or family, or consider joining a supportive community. Having a network can provide encouragement during challenging times and help maintain accountability.

3. *Overcoming Cravings and Temptations:*

- **Hydrate and Eat Balanced Meals:** Stay hydrated and consume well-balanced meals rich in fiber, protein, and healthy fats. Adequate hydration and nutrient-dense meals can help curb cravings.

- **Incorporate Treats Mindfully:** Allow occasional treats in moderation to avoid feelings of deprivation. Incorporate them mindfully into your eating plan, savoring each indulgence without derailing overall progress.

- **Identify Triggers:** Recognize emotional or situational triggers that lead to cravings. Develop alternative coping mechanisms, such as mindfulness techniques or engaging in a favorite hobby, to navigate these situations.

4. *Managing Hunger During Fasting:*

- **Stay Hydrated:** Drink water, herbal teas, or black coffee during fasting periods to stay hydrated and help manage hunger. Dehydration can sometimes be mistaken for hunger.

- **Incorporate Fiber-Rich Foods:** Include fiber-rich foods in your meals, such as vegetables and legumes, to enhance satiety. Fibre slows digestion, promoting a feeling of fullness.

- **Adjust Fasting Window:** If hunger persists, consider adjusting the fasting window. Experiment with shorter or longer fasting periods to find a balance that aligns with your energy needs and preferences.

5. *Balancing Exercise and Recovery:*

- **Prioritize Rest Days:** Integrate rest days into your exercise routine to allow for adequate recovery. Rest is crucial for muscle repair and overall well-being.

- **Adjust Intensity:** If experiencing fatigue or burnout, reassess the intensity and frequency of your workouts. Periodically incorporate lower-intensity activities or engage in active recovery exercises.

- **Listen to Your Body:** Pay attention to signs of overtraining, such as persistent fatigue, soreness, or changes in mood. Listen to your body, and adjust your exercise routine accordingly to prevent burnout.

6. *Dealing with Social and Peer Pressure:*

- **Communicate Boundaries:** Clearly communicate your health goals and boundaries to friends and family. Educate them on your chosen approach and seek their understanding and support.

- **Plan Ahead for Social Events:** Plan your approach to social events by considering the menu and potential challenges. Bring your own nutritious options or eat beforehand to maintain control over your choices.

- **Celebrate Non-Food Achievements:** Shift the focus from food-centric celebrations to non-food acheivements. Celebrate milestones with activities, experiences, or other meaniningful rewards that align with your health goals.

7. *Staying Motivated Over the Long Term:*

- **Revisit Goals:** Regularly revisit and adjust your health goals to keep them relevant and inspiring. Celebrate achievements and set new milestones to maintain a sense ofpurpose.

- **Incorporate Enjoyable Activities:** Ensure that your exercise routine includes activities you genuinely enjoy. Whether it's dancing, hiking, or playing a sport, the more enjoyable the activity, the more likely you are to stay motivated.

- **Visualize Long-Term Benefits:** Remind yourself of the long-term benefits ofyour health journey, such as improved well-being, increased energy, and reduced risk of chronic diseases. Visualizing these outcomes can reignite motivation.

8. *Seeking Professional Guidance:*

- **Consult Healthcare Professionals:** If facing persistent challenges, consult with healthcare professionals for personalized guidance. A registered dietitian, fitness trainer, or mental health professional can offer insights tailored to your unique circumstances.

• **Explore Supportive Communities:** Joining online or local communities focused on similar health goals can provide a valuable support network. Sharing experiences, challenges, and successes with others can foster motivation and resilience.

Navigating potential setbacks on your health journey requires a combination of self-awareness, flexibility, and proactive problem-solving. By troubleshooting common challenges and implementing practical solutions, you empower yourself to overcome obstacles, maintain consistency, and achieve long-term success in your pursuit of optimal health. Remember that setbacks are natural, and your ability to adapt and persevere ultimately contributes to the resilience of your health journey.

Celebrating successes and maintaining long-term health: Emphasize the sustainability of the chosen lifestyle changes and encourage ongoing healthy habits for sustained results.

Embarking on a journey to improve health through intermittent fasting, a low-carb lifestyle, and regular exercise is a commendable endeavor. As you achieve milestones and witness positive changes, it's crucial to celebrate successes and focus on the sustainability of the chosen lifestyle changes. Embracing habits that stand the test of time ensures not only short-term triumphs but also a foundation for lasting well-being. Let's explore the importance of celebrating successes and fostering ongoing healthy habits for sustained results.

1. *Reflect on Achievements:*

- **Acknowledge Milestones:** Take time to acknowledge and celebrate the achievements you've made along the way. Whether it's reaching a weight loss goal, improving blood sugar levels, or achieving new fitness milestones, recognizing your progress reinforces a positive mindset.

- **Non-Scale Victories:** Celebrate non-scale victories, such as increased energy, improved mood, or enhanced overall well-being. These qualitative changes are equally significant indicators of success.

2. *Embrace Sustainable Lifestyle Changes:*

- **Integration into Daily Life:** Ensure that intermittent fasting, a low-carb lifestyle, and exercise seamlessly integrate into your daily routine. Sustainable changes are those that become natural components of your lifestyle, allowing for long-term adherence.

- **Flexible Approaches:** Recognize the need for flexibility within your chosen lifestyle changes. Life is dynamic, and the ability to adapt your approach while maintaining the core principles ensures resilience over time.

3. *Set New Goals:*

- **Continual Progress:** Set new health and wellness goals to maintain a sense of purpose and continual progress. These goals can be both short-term and long-term, fostering a mindset of ongoing improvement.

- **Diversify Objectives:** Beyond physical goals, consider objectives related to mental and emotional well-being. Goals could include reducing stress, improving sleep quality, or enhancing mindfulness practices.

4. Enjoy the Journey:

- **Cultivate Enjoyment:** Ensure that the chosen lifestyle changes bring a sense ofjoy and fulfillment. Whether it's finding pleasure in nutritious meals, discovering new exercises you love, or savoring the benefits of intermittent fasting, a positive experience fosters sustained commitment.

- **Mindful Eating Practices**: Embrace mindful eating practices that promote a healthy relationship with food. Pay attention to hunger and fullness cues, savor flavors, and appreciate the nourishment your body receives.

5. Build a Support System:

- **Engage with Supportive Networks:** Maintain connections with supportive friends, family, or communities who share similar health goals. Sharing successes, challenges, and experiences with others creates a sense of camaraderie and reinforces motivation.

- **Professional Guidance:** If needed, continue seeking guidance from healthcare professionals, nutritionists, or fitness experts. Their expertise can provide valuable insights and adjustments as you navigate the complexities of health and well-being.

6. Prioritize Self-Care:

- **Holistic Well-Being:** Prioritize holistic well-being by incorporating self-care practices into your routine. Adequate sleep, stress management, and activities that bring joy contribute to overall health and resilience.

- **Rest and Recovery:** Recognize the importance of rest and recovery, both in terms of exercise and daily life. Balanced routines that include periods of rest ensure sustainability and prevent burnout.

7. Foster a Positive Mindset:

- **Gratitude Practice:** Cultivate a gratitude practice by acknowledging the positive aspects of your health journey. Gratitude reinforces a positive mindset, fostering resilience during challenging times.

- **Positive Affirmations:** Use positive affirmations to reinforce your commitment to long-term health. Remind yourself of the progress made and the positive impact your chosen lifestyle changes have on your life.

8. Periodic Assessments and Adjustments:

- **Reassess and Adapt:** Periodically reassess your goals, preferences, and health status. Adapt your approach as needed to align with your evolving needs and circumstances.

- **Celebrate Continuous Improvement:** Embrace the concept of continuous improvement rather than perfection. Celebrate the journey of becoming the healthiest version of yourself overtime.

9. Educate and Empower Yourself:

- **Stay Informed:** Continue educating yourself on the latest research and insights related to intermittent fasting, low-carb living, and exercise. Knowledge empowers you to make informed choices that align with your health goals.

• **Personalize Your Approach**: Understand that everyone's health journey is unique. Personalize your approach based on your individual preferences, health status, and responses to lifestyle changes.

Celebrating successes and maintaining long-term health is an ongoing process that requires commitment, adaptability, and a positive mindset. By emphasizing the sustainability of lifestyle changes and fostering habits that align with your well-being, you create a foundation for lasting results. As you navigate the journey towards optimal health, remember that every positive choice contributes to your overall well-being, and the path to sustained health is a lifelong adventure worth embracing.

Conclusion

In conclusion, "Revitalize Your Health: A Comprehensive Guide to Weight Loss and Type 2 Diabetes Reversal through Intermittent Fasting and Low Carb Living" serves as a roadmap for individuals seeking transformative changes in their well-being. This comprehensive guide has explored the intricate interplay between intermittent fasting, adopting a low-carb lifestyle, and incorporating regular exercise as powerful tools in achieving sustainable weight loss and potentially reversing Type 2 diabetes.

The journey towards optimal health is not just about shedding pounds but embracing a holistic lifestyle that fosters long-term vitality. By understanding the intricacies of Type 2 diabetes, exploring the benefits of intermittent fasting, and delving into the nuances of a low-carb lifestyle, readers are equipped with the knowledge to make informed choices for their health.

The guide emphasizes the importance of celebrating successes, acknowledging milestones, and maintaining a positive mindset throughout the health journey. It underscores the need for sustainable lifestyle changes that seamlessly integrate into daily life, ensuring adherence and resilience over time.

As readers navigate potential setbacks and challenges, the guide provides practical solutions, encouraging adaptability and a proactive approach to overcoming obstacles. By monitoring progress through various indicators such as weight, blood sugar levels, and overall well-being, individuals can make informed adjustments, fostering a dynamic and personalized health plan.

The journey toward optimal health is not a one-size-fits-all endeavor. It requires continual self-assessment, periodic goal-setting, and an openness to evolving strategies. The guide concludes by emphasizing the significance of long-term commitment, self-care practices, and ongoing education to stay informed and empowered on the path to sustained well-being.

"Revitalize Your Health" is more than a guide; it is an invitation to embrace a transformative lifestyle—one that revitalizes not just the body but the spirit. As individuals embark on this holistic journey, they are encouraged to celebrate every achievement, learn from setbacks, and revel in the ongoing process of becoming the healthiest version of themselves. May this guide serve as a beacon of empowerment and inspiration, guiding individuals toward a revitalized and flourishing life.